VANDANA KAPOOR

HOME REMIDIES

Natural Solutions for Everyday Wellness

Copyright © 2024 by Vandana Kapoor

All rights reserved. No part of this publication may be reproduced, stored or transmitted in any form or by any means, electronic, mechanical, photocopying, recording, scanning, or otherwise without written permission from the publisher. It is illegal to copy this book, post it to a website, or distribute it by any other means without permission.

Vandana Kapoor asserts the moral right to be identified as the author of this work.

Vandana Kapoor has no responsibility for the persistence or accuracy of URLs for external or third-party Internet Websites referred to in this publication and does not guarantee that any content on such Websites is, or will remain, accurate or appropriate.

Designations used by companies to distinguish their products are often claimed as trademarks. All brand names and product names used in this book and on its cover are trade names, service marks, trademarks and registered trademarks of their respective owners. The publishers and the book are not associated with any product or vendor mentioned in this book. None of the companies referenced within the book have endorsed the book.

First edition

This book was professionally typeset on Reedsy.
Find out more at reedsy.com

This book is dedicated to the vibrant and curious spirits of the younger generation. Here's to embracing a journey of self-care and holistic living.

The greatest remedies are found in the
simplest places.

VANDY

Contents

1

Introduction:

In a world where quick fixes and pharmaceutical solutions often take center stage, "Home Remedies: Natural Solutions for Everyday Wellness" offers a refreshing return to nature's bounty. This book has been crafted with the purpose of reintroducing the timeless wisdom of simple, natural remedies that have been trusted across cultures and generations.This book has born out of a deep concern for the rising health challenges faced by young people today – challenges amplified by the stress of modern living and prolonged screen time that often disconnects us from the healing embrace of Mother Nature. Our young generation is navigating a world where the boundaries between work, study, and personal life are increasingly blurred, resulting in heightened stress levels and a host of related health issues. From sleep disturbances to anxiety, from chronic headaches to digestive discomforts, the physical and mental toll is evident. Compounded with this is the digital era's impact, where hours spent in front of screens are not just a part of leisure but a necessity for education and professional commitments, leading to a disconnect from the natural world and its intrinsic healing properties.

I genuinely hope that this book strikes a chord with the younger generation, encouraging them to invest a little time in exploring these straightforward remedies. After all, they have nothing to lose and potentially a great deal to gain in terms of health and well-being.

2

Inspiration:

Our ancestors relied on the healing properties of herbs, spices, and common household ingredients long before modern medicine came into existence. This book aims to bridge the gap between ancient knowledge and contemporary living, providing easy-to-follow, effective remedies for common ailments, wellness, and overall health maintenance.

At its core "Home Remedies" is more than just a compilation of natural treatments. It is a testament to the power of nature in promoting healing and well-being, and an invitation to explore a more holistic approach to health. Each remedy in this book is carefully selected for its effectiveness, ease of preparation, accessibility of ingredients.

Furthermore, this book serves as an empowering tool, encouraging readers to take an active role in their health and well-being. It is about rediscovering the joy of creating your own natural treatments and experiencing the satisfaction of self-care.

This book reconnects you with simple benefits of Mother

Nature's gifts.

As I embark on sharing the wisdom encapsulated in this book of "Home Remedies: Natural Solutions for Everyday Wellness," my mind wanders back to the warm, comforting kitchen of my grandmother. It was a magical place where ailments met their match in the form of herbal concoctions, soothing syrups, and age-old wisdom. This book is a tribute to those times – a compilation of simple yet effective remedies passed down through generations in my family, seasoned with love and care.

Growing up, our home was a sanctuary where the common cold, flu, and other everyday illnesses were treated not just with medicine, but with a generous dose of nurturing and natural remedies. Our grandmother, a repository of traditional knowledge, believed firmly in the healing powers of nature. Her kitchen was her apothecary, filled with the aroma of herbs and spices, where each jar and bottle held remedies steeped in history and tradition.

In these pages, I share with you the remedies that were a staple in our home. From the ginger tea that soothed a sore throat to the turmeric milk that was the antidote to a cold, each recipe is a piece of my childhood These remedies are more than just treatments for physical ailments; they are memories of the care and love that went into preparing them.

This book is not just a collection of home remedies; it is a journey through the lanes of memory, a testament to the wisdom of our mothers and grandmothers, and an invitation to embrace the natural way of healing. It reflects a time when healthcare was as much about the warmth of a hug and the comfort of a home-cooked meal as it was about healing. This book covers home remedies which are for ailments like, insomnia, constipation, headaches, stress, anxiety toothaches, throat aches, cough, cold, fever, acne, colicky babies, arthritis, depression, burns and many more ailments. This will help you to tackle common ailments by using things available at your home.

You must have heard of Newton's Third Law of Motion: "Every action in nature there is an equal and opposite reaction." This clearly means any medicine we consume, our bodies will surely have a reaction in some other part of our body.

Did you Know which countries spends most on medicines?

Compared with other high-income countries, the United States spends the most

per-capital income on prescription drugs, followed by Germany, Canada, Korea, and the list goes on.

Once you read this book and start using these remedies you will feel that you have a doctor available to you and to your friends and family 24*7.

The remedies shared in this book are as old as Ayurveda, and have been passed generation after generation and I wish to share it with my newly acquired family through this book. We will divulge in two kinds of remedies, one for minor ailments and the other for household rectification remedies. Before we go on any further discussing the remedies, please read the below Disclaimer.

Please Note:

Disclaimer: Since you are dealing with health-related content, it is important to note that these remedies are not substitutes for medical advice.

3

Simple Solutions for Everyday Ailments

INSOMNIA:

Ingredients: Lavender oil, Chamomile tea leaves or tea bag.

- ·Before going to bed take nice hot shower and rub Lavender oil on your palms of your hands and under your feet for 5 minutes each and then sip Chamomile tea.
- Deep Breathing for 5 minutes, 6 times a day for 2-3 minutes each time.
- Exercise during the day.

STRESS & ANXIETY:

- Meditation before bed is excellent for sleep. Cuddle any family member, friends, or any pet.
- Exercise- concentrating on breathing exercises.
- Reduce Caffeine intake.
- No alcohol.

COLD:

Ingredients: Honey, ginger, garlic, leafy vegetables, salt.

- Boil water and let the ginger steep in the water then add tea without milk and add honey in it.
- Increase garlic intake in your food.
- Put two drops saline water in each of your nostrils.
- Have food rich in Vitamin C, like green leafy vegetables, citrus fruits.
- Can put essential oils like Tea tree, Eucalyptus, Thyme, and Menthol while taking a bath, this helps.

SORE THROAT:

Ingredients: Pepper, ginger, basil, honey, salt, turmeric, marsh mellows.

- Take a glass of water add 4 pods of pepper, some ginger, cloves and 6 leaves of Basil, boil till the water becomes half, divide this into three portions and have three times a day. You can add honey in each portion before you have.
- Do saline gargles three to four times a day.
- Take some tea leaves and boil in water, let it become Luke warm and then gargle with it three times a day.
- You can also gargle with Turmeric, it is very effective, it has a compound called cur cumin works like an antiseptic and tackles any infection in the respiratory tracts.
- Add three to four marshmallows to soothe a sore throat. The gelatin in the marshmallows is what soothes the sore throat.

TOOTHACHE:

Ingredients; Salt, wheat grass, clove oil, vanilla extract, garlic paste

- Rinse area of effected tooth by salt water or wheat grass, apply clove oil, vanilla extract or garlic paste.
- Apply a cold compression of ice to the affected area.

CONSTIPATION:

Ingredients: Caffeinated coffee, prunes, figs, raisins, Aloe Vera juice

·Drink coffee- only caffeinated one.

·Soak 4 prunes/figs overnight and have the water and the prunes in the morning.

·Have 7-8 raisins during the day.

·Avoid dairy products.

·Have warm water.

·Aloe Vera juice is good too.

·Sit in a squat position.

ARTHRITIS:

Ingredients: Salt, probiotic yogurt, honey, turmeric, garlic, ginger.

- Have a nice warm salt bath.
- Have probiotic yogurt and mix 2 spoons of organic honey and have every day to reduce pain in joints.
- Have half teaspoon of turmeric (cur cumin) every day in the morning.
- Have a pod of garlic either in the morning or at bed time, for 8 weeks at least.
- Have ginger in food or in any form of teas for 12 weeks at

least.
- Use Paraffin wax to soothe joint pain and stiffness, melt the paraffin wax in a wax heater, clean the area you want to apply it at, check the temperature of the wax and then apply, wrap the area with a plastic or silver foil for 30 minutes, the warm wax gives heat and lubrication to the joints and reduces inflammation.

FEVER:

Ingredients: Broth, ginger, garlic, turmeric, ice, honey.

- Have plenty of broth-based soups and include ginger, garlic, and turmeric in it.
- Suck on ice if fever is high.
- Do cold compression taking a hand towel and putting it in your forehead, back of neck and under your feet.
- Have a tea with ginger and honey two to three times a day.

COLICKY BABIES:

Ingredients; Asafoetida, warm towel.

- Make them lie down on their tummy's.
- Put a warm towel over the babies naval.
- Rub a pinch of Asafoetida on the babies naval.

CUTS AND BRUISES:

Ingredients: Soap, Honey, Aloe Vera, Turmeric paste, Tea bags.

- Rinse the cut with cool running water to remove dirt and debris.

- Gently clean the area with mild soap and water.
- **Apply Pressure:** For bleeding cuts, apply gentle pressure with a clean cloth or sterile bandage to control bleeding.
- **Honey:**Apply a thin layer of raw honey to the wound. Honey has antibacterial properties and can promote healing.
- **Aloe Vera:** Use fresh aloe Vera gel or ointment on the cut or bruise for its soothing and anti-inflammatory effects.
- **Turmeric Paste:**Mix turmeric powder with a small amount of water to form a paste.
- Apply the paste to the bruised area for its anti-inflammatory properties.
- **Tea Bags:**Place cooled tea bags (such as black or green tea) on bruises to help reduce discoloration.

BURNS:

Ingredients: Cold milk, Aloe Vera, honey, coconut oil, cucumber, potato, avocado.

- Wash the burned area with cool water or cold milk.
- Apply Aloe Vera on the burns.
- Apply honey on the burns.
- Then apply coconut oil on the affected area.
- Use a cool wet tea bag on the area of burns.
- Apply cucumber or potato slices.
- Mash Avocado and apply on the burn and let it dry.

FEVER BLISTERS:

Ingredients: Petroleum Jelly.

- Apply petroleum jelly to the skin.

- Apply cold compress on the affected area.
- Avoid eating nuts and chocolate.

NAIL FUNGUS:

Nail fungus, also known as onychomycosis, can be persistent, but there are several home remedies that may help manage and improve the condition. It is important to note that results can vary, and severe cases may require professional medical attention. Here are some common home remedies for nail fungus:

- **Tea Tree Oil:**
- Apply tea tree oil directly to the affected nails using a cotton ball. Tea tree oil has anti fungal properties that may help combat nail fungus.
- **Vinegar Soak:**
- Soak your affected nails in a mixture of equal parts white vinegar and warm water for about 15-20 minutes daily. Dry thoroughly afterward.
- **Listerine Soak:**
- Soak your nails in a mixture of Listerine mouthwash and warm water for about 15-20 minutes daily. Listerine contains anti fungal properties.
- **Garlic:**
- Crush garlic cloves and apply the paste directly to the affected nails. Garlic has natural anti fungal properties.
- **Baking Soda Paste:**
- Mix baking soda with water to create a paste. Apply the paste to the affected nails and leave it on for 10-15 minutes before rinsing.
- **Hydrogen Peroxide Soak:**

- Soak your affected nails in a mixture of hydrogen peroxide and warm water for about 15 minutes. Dry thoroughly afterward.

HEARTBURN:
Ingredients: Baking soda, bananas, ginger,white pepper.

- Dissolve a tsp. of baking soda in 8 ounces (1 cup) of water and drink. Baking soda is a natural antacid.
- Banana's act as a natural antacid in the body. You can eat either fresh or dried bananas.
- Fresh ginger is one of the oldest remedies for heartburn. It can be added t to food when its cooked, eaten raw, or consumed as ginger tea.
- Chew 4 pods of white pepper ,this will decrease the heartburn immediately (have tried this myself and it works wonderfully).

UPSET STOMATCH:
Ingredients: Ginger, rice, crackers, bananas, peppermint.

- Ginger tea or ginger ale can help with nausea.
- Eat bland foods like crackers, rice, and bananas.
- Peppermint tea may help soothe an upset stomach

LICE TREATMENT:
Dealing with head lice can be challenging, but there are several home remedies that may help in the treatment and prevention of lice infestations.

- **Tea Tree Oil:**
- Mix a few drops of tea tree oil with a carrier oil (such as coconut oil) and apply it to the scalp. Leave it on for a few hours or overnight, then comb through the hair with a fine-toothed comb to remove dead lice and nits.
- **Mayonnaise or Olive Oil:**
- Coat the hair and scalp with mayonnaise or olive oil, cover it with a shower cap, and leave it on overnight. Wash the hair thoroughly the next morning and comb out the dead lice and nits.
- **VINEGAR:**
- Apply white vinegar to the hair and scalp, cover with a shower cap, and leave it on for a few hours. Rinse the hair thoroughly and comb out the lice and nits.
- **SALT:**
- Mix salt with vinegar to create a paste. Apply the paste to the scalp and leave it on for a few hours. Wash the hair and comb out the lice and nits.
- **GARLIC:**
- Make a paste by crushing garlic cloves and mix it with lime juice. Apply the paste to the scalp, leave it on for 30 minutes, and then wash the hair.
- **PETROLEUM JELLY:**
- Apply petroleum jelly to the scalp and hair, cover it with a shower cap, and leave it on overnight. Wash the hair thoroughly the next morning and comb out the lice and nits.
- **ONION JUICE:**
- Extract onion juice and apply it to the scalp. Leave it on for a few hours before washing the hair.

<u>REMEDIES FOR EYES:</u>

- **Warm Compress:**
- Use a warm compress on your eyes to reduce eye strain and soothe tired eyes.
- Simply soak a clean cloth in warm water, wring it out, and place it over closed eyes for a few minutes.
- **Cucumber Slices:**
- Place chilled cucumber slices on your closed eyes for about 10-15 minutes.
- Cucumbers have a cooling effect and may help reduce puffiness.
- **Tea Bags:**
- Place steeped and cooled tea bags (especially chamomile or green tea) on closed eyes for 15 minutes.
- Tea bags contain antioxidants that may help soothe irritated eyes.
- **Cold Compress for Puffy Eye:**
- Use a cold compress or ice pack wrapped in a thin cloth to reduce puffiness around the eyes.
- Apply it for 5-10 minutes.
- **Eye Exercises:**
- Practice eye exercises to reduce eye strain and improve focus.
- Rotate your eyes clockwise and counterclockwise, and focus on objects at different distances.
- **Rosewater:**
- Soak a cotton ball with rosewater and apply over the eyelids.
- Rosewater is known for its soothing properties.

4

Beauty Maintenance Unveiled

R<u>EMEDIES FOR WHITENING TEETH:</u>

- **Baking Soda and Hydrogen Peroxide**
- **Ingredients: Baking Soda and Hydrogen Peroxide**
  - Make a paste by mixing baking soda with hydrogen peroxide.
  - Brush your teeth with this paste, but do this sparingly as excessive use may damage enamel.

  -

  - **Strawberries and Baking Soda**
  - **Ingredients: Strawberries, Baking Soda**
  - Mash strawberries and mix with baking soda to form a paste.
  - Apply the paste to your teeth for a few minutes before brushing.

- **Apple Cider Vinegar**
- **Ingredients: Apple Cider Vinegar and Water**
- Gargle with a diluted solution of apple cider vinegar and water.
- Rinse your mouth thoroughly afterward as is acidic and may erode enamel.

- **Turmeric Powder**
- **Ingredients: Turmeric and Water.**
- Make a paste using turmeric powder and water.
- Apply the paste to your teeth and leave it on for a few minutes before rinsing.

- **Dietary Adjustments**
- Limit the consumption of wine and dark colored food and beverages like coffee, chocolate, tea.
- Increase the intake of crunchy fruits and vegetables like apples, celery etc.

REMEDIES FOR FACE GLOW:

- The most important thing to do for your skin is to have plenty of water so that your skin can remain hydrated from inside.
- Daily exercise is a must with a healthy diet.
- Adequate sleep.

- Use a Sun Screen SPF 30 minimum, before you step out.

- **Exfoliation**
- **Ingredients: Oatmeal, Sugar, and Honey.**
- Regular exfoliation helps remove dead skin cells, promoting a brighter complexion.
- Use a gentle exfoliating scrub or consider oatmeal or sugar mixed with honey which acts an exfoliating agent.

- **Honey and Lemon Mask**
- **Ingredients: Honey and Lemon.**
- Mix honey with a few drops of lemon juice.
- Apply the mixture to your face and leave it on for about 15 minutes before rinsing off.

- **Yogurt Mask**
- **Ingredients: Yogurt**
- Apply plain yogurt to your face and leave it on for 15-20 minutes.
- The lactic acid in yogurt can help exfoliate and hydrate the skin.

- **Turmeric and Honey Face Mask (one of my favorites)**

- **Ingredients: Turmeric and Honey**
- Mix turmeric powder with yogurt or honey to form a paste.
- Apply the paste to your face, leave it on for 15 minutes, and then rinse off.

- **Aloe Vera Gel**
- **Ingredients: Aloe Vera Gel or if you have fresh Aloe Vera plant**
- Apply fresh Aloe Vera gel on your face, if you have an Aloe Vera plant, then cut the leaf remove the small thorns from the sides and peel the skin from one side, keep in the refrigerator for 15 min before applying.
- Aloe Vera has soothing and moisturizing properties that can contribute to a healthy glow.

- **Rosewater**
- Use rosewater as a toner to refresh and hydrate your skin.
- You can also mix rosewater with glycerin for added moisture.

- **Cucumber**
- Place chilled cucumber slices on your eyes and rub your face with it for a refreshing effect.
- Cucumber can help reduce puffiness around your eyes and soothes the skin.

<u>ACNE:</u>

- Gently wash your face twice daily using a mild, fragrance-free cleanser. Avoid scrubbing vigorously, as it can irritate the skin.Use any of these remedies for a week to see the difference.
- **Tea Tree Oil:**
- Apply diluted tea tree oil to acne-prone areas. Tea tree oil has antimicrobial properties that may help reduce acne lesions.
- **Honey and Cinnamon Mask:**
- Mix honey and cinnamon to create a paste. Apply the mixture to affected areas, leave it on for 10-15 minutes, and then rinse.
- **Aloe Vera Gel:**
- Apply fresh aloe Vera gel to acne-prone skin. Aloe Vera has anti-inflammatory and soothing properties.
- **Apple Cider Vinegar Toner:**
- Dilute apple cider vinegar with water (1:1 ratio) and use it as a toner. Start with a patch test, and if well-tolerated, apply to the face using a cotton pad.
- **Green Tea:**
- Apply cooled, brewed green tea to the skin using a cotton ball. Green tea contains antioxidants with potential anti-inflammatory effects.
- **Ice Cube:**
- Wrap an ice cube in a thin cloth and apply it to the affected area for a few minutes to reduce inflammation and soothe the skin.
- **Turmeric Paste:**
- Mix turmeric powder with water or yogurt to create a paste.

Apply it to the acne-prone areas and leave it on for 15 minutes before rinsing.

- **Baking Soda Exfoliation:**
- Create a paste with baking soda and water. Gently exfoliate your skin with the mixture, but use caution as it can be abrasive.

REMEDIES TO MAINTAIN HEALTHY HAIR:

Coconut Oil Massage

- Warm coconut oil and massage it into your scalp.
- Leave it on for at least 30 minutes or overnight, then shampoo as usual.
- Coconut oil helps nourish the hair and may improve its overall health.

Egg Mask

- Beat an egg and apply it to your hair.
- Leave it on for about 20 minutes before washing it out.
- Eggs are rich in protein, which can strengthen hair.

Aloe Vera Treatment

- Apply fresh aloe Vera gel to your scalp and hair.
- Leave it on for 30 minutes before rinsing.
- Aloe Vera can soothe the scalp and promote healthy hair growth.

Avocado Hair Mask

- Mash a ripe avocado and apply it to damp hair.
- Leave it on for 20-30 minutes before rinsing.
- Avocado is rich in vitamins and healthy fats, promoting shiny hair.

Yogurt Hair Mask

- Mix yogurt with a tablespoon of honey and apply it to your hair.
- Leave it on for 20-30 minutes before rinsing.
- Yogurt can provide nourishment, and honey adds moisture.

Banana Hair Mask

- Mash a ripe banana and mix it with yogurt.
- Apply the mixture to your hair and leave it on for 30 minutes before washing.
- Bananas are rich in vitamins and can add moisture to your hair.

Onion Juice For Hair Growth (My favorite as I have tried it personally)

- ·Extract onion juice and apply it to your scalp.
- ·Leave it on for 30 minutes before washing your hair.
- Onion juice is believed to stimulate hair follicles and promote hair growth.

Remember to test these remedies on a small patch of skin to ensure you do not have any adverse reactions. If you have specific concerns about your hair or scalp, it is advisable to consult with a dermatologist or a healthcare professional for personalized advice.

DANDRUFF:

Dealing with dandruff can be bothersome, but there are several home remedies that may help manage and reduce its symptoms. Here are some common and natural remedies for dandruff:

- **Tea Tree Oil:**
- Add a few drops of tea tree oil to your regular shampoo and use it when washing your hair. Tea tree oil has anti fungal properties that may help reduce dandruff.
- **Coconut Oil:**
- Massage warm coconut oil into your scalp and leave it on for at least 30 minutes before washing your hair. Coconut oil can moisturize the scalp and reduce dandruff.
- **Aloe Vera:**
- Apply fresh aloe Vera gel directly to the scalp. Aloe Vera has soothing and anti-inflammatory properties that may help with dandruff.
- **Apple Cider Vinegar Rinse:**
- Mix equal parts apple cider vinegar and water. Use this mixture as a final rinse after shampooing. It can help balance the PH of the scalp and reduce dandruff.
- **Baking Soda Scrub:**
- Wet your hair, then rub a handful of baking soda into your scalp. Rinse thoroughly. Baking soda can help exfoliate the scalp and reduce flakes.
- **Lemon Juice:**

- Massage fresh lemon juice into your scalp and leave it on for a few minutes before washing your hair. Lemon juice has antimicrobial properties that may help with dandruff.
- **Yogurt Hair Mask:**
- Apply plain yogurt to your scalp and leave it on for about 15-20 minutes before washing your hair. Yogurt can provide relief from dandruff and nourish the scalp.
- **Neem Oil:**(other names for which include Azadirachta indica and Indian lilac)
- Mix neem oil with a carrier oil (like coconut or jojoba oil) and massage it into your scalp. Neem oil has antibacterial and anti fungal properties.
- **Onion Juice: (My Favorite)**
- Extract onion juice and apply it to your scalp. Leave it on for 30 minutes before washing. Onion juice is believed to have anti fungal properties.

REMEDIES FOR CRACKED HEEL AND FEET:

Cracked heels can be uncomfortable and unsightly, but there are several home remedies you can try to help soften and heal them. Consistent care is essential to see improvements. Here are some remedies for cracked heels:

- **Warm Water Soak**
- Soak your feet in warm, soapy water for 15-20 minutes to soften the skin.
- Use a pumice stone or foot file to gently exfoliate the dead skin.
- **Vaseline /Petroleum Jelly**
- Apply a thick layer of Vaseline or petroleum jelly to your

heels.

- Cover your feet with socks and leave it on overnight.
- This is very effective I have used this personally and within two days of using this the feet become 75% better.
- **Paraffin Wax Treatment**
- Melt paraffin wax and mix it with coconut oil.
- Apply the mixture to your feet, let it cool, and then peel it off
- This too is very effective; I have used this personally.\

5

Quick Fixes to Household Woes

S*TAINS:*
You could stain your clothes by dropping coffee, tea, grease from food, wine, ink, blood etc.

Here are some quick fixes for you.

Act quickly: The sooner you address a stain, the better the chances of successful removal.

- Blot, do not rub: Gently blot the stain with a clean cloth or paper towel to avoid spreading it.

Coffee or Tea Stains

- Rinse the stain with cold water immediately
- Pr-treat with a mixture of vinegar and water or a mild dish soap.
- Launder as usual.

Wine Stains

- Blot the stain with a clean cloth.
- Sprinkle salt or baking soda on the stain to absorb excess liquid.
- Rinse with cold water, then launder.

Ink Stains

- Place a paper towel under the stained area.
- Dab the stain with rubbing alcohol using a cotton ball.
- Launder as usual.

Grease /Oil Stains

- Blot excess oil with a paper towel.
- Apply a small amount of dish soap or liquid laundry detergent to the stain.
- Wash in the hottest water suitable for the fabric.

Blood Stains

- Rinse the stain with cold water as soon as possible.
- Soak the garment in cold water with salt or enzyme-based stain remover.
- Launder as usual.
- **<u>Additional Tips</u>**
- Vinegar: White vinegar can be used for many stains. Mix with water and blot or apply to the stain.
- Lemon Juice: Lemon juice can be effective on some stains. Sunlight may enhance its stain-removing properties
- Hydrogen Peroxide: Diluted hydrogen peroxide can be applied to certain stains, but test in an inconspicuous area

first.

CAUTION

Always check care labels on your clothing for specific instructions.

Avoid using hot water on protein-based stains like blood, as it can set the stain.

Test any stain remover on a small, inconspicuous area first to ensure it will not damage the fabric.

ODOR REMOVAL:

- There can be several types of Odors which bother us in our homes like Odors from the refrigerator, Odors from the garbage, form the dish washing area, from the microwave, from the clogged drains.
- Odor removal is a common household concern, and there are several effective and natural solutions to tackle unwanted smells.

Refrigerator Odors:

Place an open box of baking soda in the refrigerator to absorb unwanted Odors.

Garbage Disposal Odor:

Grind citrus peels in the disposal to freshen it up.

Microwave Odors:

Microwave a bowl of water with lemon slices for a few minutes to eliminate Odors.

Shoe Odor:

Place dry tea bags or baking soda inside shoes to absorb the Odor, please make sure that the shoes are dry before using this method.

CLOGGED DRAINS:

- Sometimes we need immediate attention from clogged drains and the plumber is not easily available, for such situations we have simple remedies like;
- Pour a mixture of baking soda and vinegar down the drain, followed by hot water, to help clear minor clogs.
- For preventive maintenance, regularly flush drains with boiling water.

FURNITURE POLISH:

Have people coming over and your furniture is looking shabby, no worries we have a quick fix for you.

- Mix equal parts olive oil and lemon juice to create a natural furniture polish.
- Apply the mixture with a soft cloth for a shiny finish.

PET STAINS:

- Mix white vinegar with water and blot pet stains on carpets or upholstery.
- Sprinkle baking soda on the affected area, let it sit, and then vacuum.

INSECT REPELLENT:

- Place cucumber slices or lemon peels at entry points to deter ants.

- Use a mixture of water and vinegar as a natural insect repellent.

STICKER RESIDUE REMOVER:

Apply a small amount of cooking oil to sticker residue and let it sit for a few minutes before wiping away.

CRAYON MARKS ON WALLS:

We all have children in the house and we know how inquisitive and impatient they are, many a times we must deal with our children painting on walls and then we try and scrub the walls leaving bigger stains on the walls, here is a very easy and simple remedy for removing crayon marks from the walls.

- Gently rub toothpaste on crayon marks on walls, then wipe with a damp cloth.

RUST REMOVAL:

- Make a paste with lemon juice and salt and apply it to rust stains. Let it sit, then scrub and rinse.

SILVER POLISH:

- Create a paste using baking soda and water to polish silverware. Apply, rub gently, and then rinse.

DUSTY LAMPSHADES:

- Use a lint roller to quickly remove dust from lampshades.

LIMESCALE REMOVER:

- Soak faucets or shower heads in white vinegar to remove limescale. Scrub with an old toothbrush and rinse.

SCORCHED PAN:

- Boil a mixture of water and baking soda in a scorched pan to loosen burnt-on food. Scrub and rinse. Cleanup.

STICKER RESIDUE ON GLASS:
Apply cooking oil or mayonnaise to sticker residue on glass surfaces, let it sit, then wipe away.

TARNISHED BRASS OR COPPER:

- Make a paste with lemon juice and salt, apply it to tarnished brass or copper, let it sit, and then buff with a cloth.

CANDLE WAX REMOVER:

- To remove melted candle wax from surfaces, place a brown paper bag over the wax and iron over it. The wax will transfer to the paper.

SHINY STAINLESS STEEL:

- Polish stainless-steel surfaces with a small amount of olive oil or baby oil to remove fingerprints and add shine.

SQUEAKY DOOR HINGES:

- Apply a small amount of petroleum jelly or cooking oil to lubricate squeaky door hinges.

CARPET DEODORIZER:

- Sprinkle baking soda on carpets before vacuuming to neutralize Odors.

MOLD AND MILDEW PREVENTION IN BATHROOMS:

- Wipe bathroom surfaces with a vinegar and water solution to prevent Mold and mildew growth.

SOME GENERAL REMEDIES:

- Use duct tape to remove warts.
- Cure nail fungus with vapor rub.
- Soothe eczema by using oatmeal
- Cure bad breath by eating yogurt.
- A spoonful of sugar to cure the hiccups.
- Bite a pencil to cure a headache.
- Eat olives to help with motion sickness

6

Home Remedy Kit

Now let us put everything together and work towards making a Home Remedy Kit. A treasure trove of natural ingredients and tools that will prepare you to handle common ailments with ease and confidence. Think of it as your personal health toolkit, tailored to meet the everyday wellness needs of you and your family.

Essentials for Your Kit:

Herbs and Spices:

- **Ginger:** Great for digestive issues, sore throats, colds, and fever.
- **Turmeric:** Known for its anti-inflammatory properties.

- **Cinnamon:** Helpful in regulating blood sugar and improving digestion.
- **Garlic:** Recognized for its immune -boosting capabilities.

33

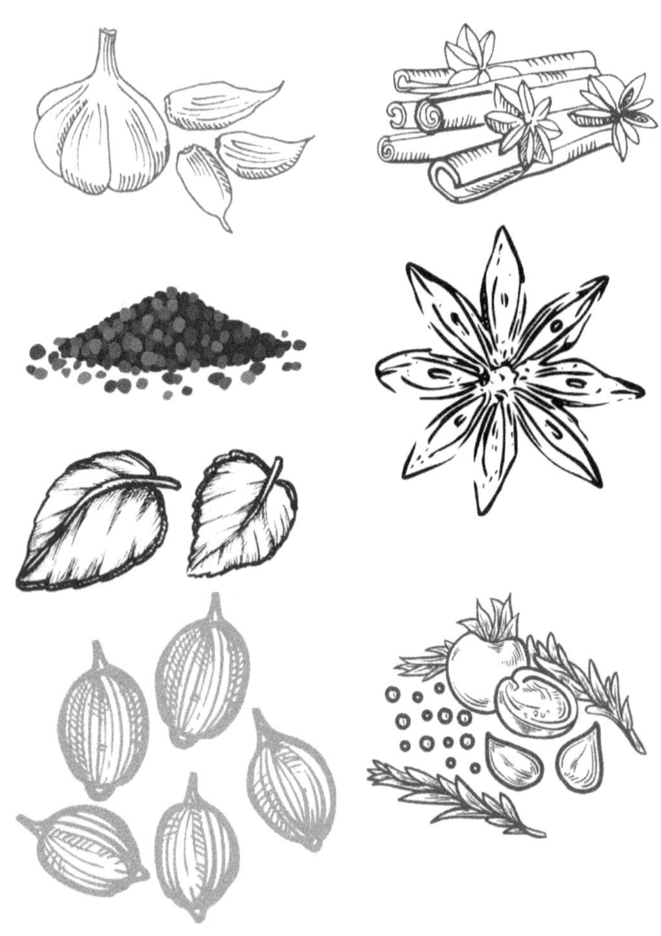

Natural Oils:

- **Coconut Oil:** Useful for skin and Hair care.

- **Eucalyptus Oil:** Excellent for respiratory issues.
- **Tea Tree Oil:** Has very good antiseptic properties.

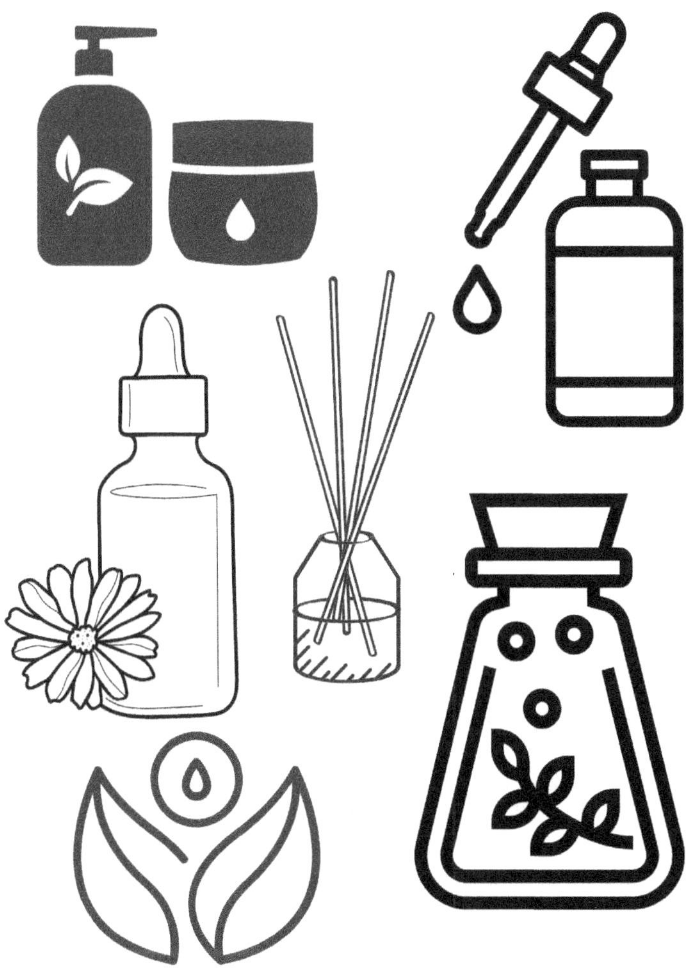

<u>Other Natural Ingredients:</u>

- **Lemon**: High on citric content and used in fever, sore throat, and many household remedies, like stain removal.
- **Honey:** Versatile use in promoting health, soothing sore throat, healing wounds, burns.
- **Aloe Vera:** Good for overall skin health, it smooth ens burns and irritable skin.
- **Apple Cider Vinegar**: Helps with digestion and sore throats.

Basic Supplies:

- Measuring cups and spoons.
- Mortar and Pestle for grinding herbs and spices.
- Jars and bottles to store homemade remedies.
- Tea Infuser for making Herbal teas.

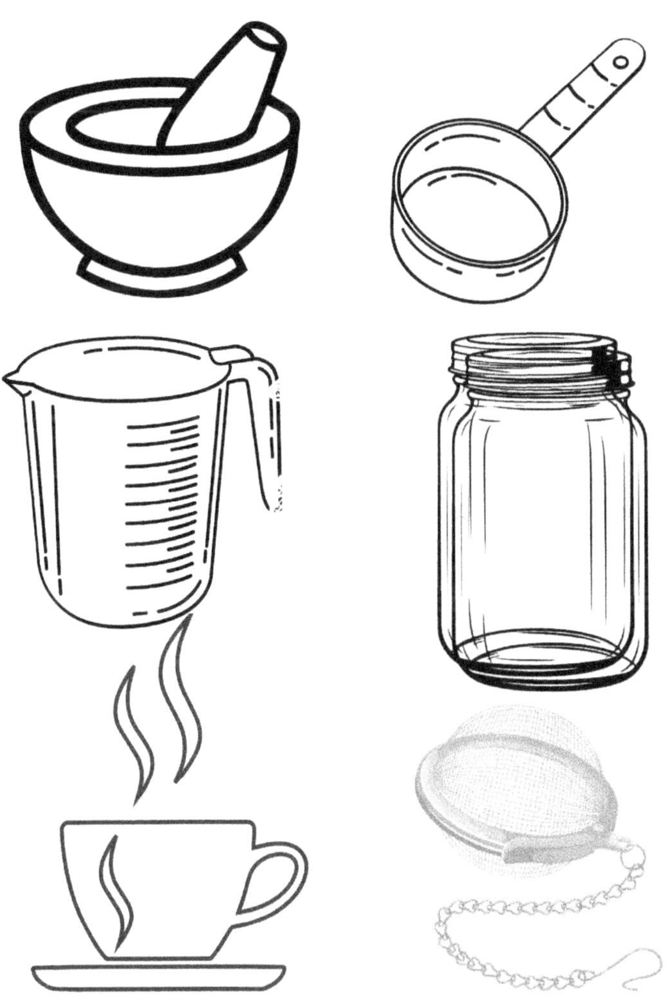

Reference Material:

- A small note book to jot down recipes.

- Books or guides on home remedies and natural healing.

<u>Safety Items:</u>

- First Aid Basics: Band-aids, sterile gauze, antiseptic wipes, thermometer.

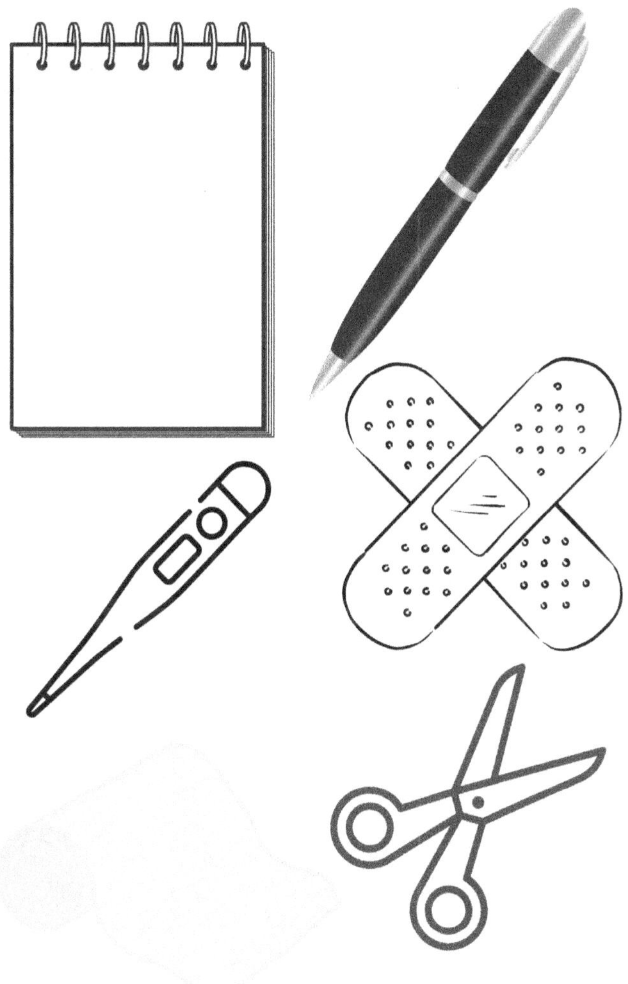

Organizing Your Kit:

Plan out how to store these items and label each home remedy with date, usage, and instructions.

Maintenance Tips:

Provide advice on regularly checking the kit for expired items, replenishing supplies, and keeping the kit in a cool, dry place.

42

7

Conclusion

In concluding this home remedies book, I want to express my sincere dedication to providing you with a collection of simple yet effective solutions for common concerns.I have poured my best efforts into compiling this resource, hoping it serves as a handy guide for promoting well-being. I trust this book enriches your understanding of home remedies and empowers you with accessible tools for a healthier lifestyle. Thank you for allowing me to be a part of your wellness journey.

DISCLAIMER:

This information is for reference purposes only and should not be considered a substitute for professional medical advice. Consult your healthcare provider before trying any home remedies, especially if you have per-existing health conditions or concerns. Individual responses may vary, and it is essential to perform patch tests to avoid allergic reactions. If adverse effects occur, discontinue use, and seek advice. Home remedies are not

a replacement for proper medical care, and any delay in seeking professional attention is not recommended.

If 'Natural Solutions for Everyday Wellness' has become trusted companion in your journey to holistic well-being, I invite you to share your experience. Your thoughts matter greatly, **and by leaving a review**, you are not only expressing your appreciation but also guiding others toward a path of natural remedies and a healthier lifestyle. Thank you for being a part of this wellness exploration. Your feedback is invaluable.

8

Resources

https://www.medicalnewstoday.com/articles/318694#avoid-dairy

13 home remedies for constipation. (2024, January 19). https://www.medicalnewstoday.com/articles/318694#avoid-dairy

https://www.healthline.com/health/osteoarthritis/arthritis-natural-relief#diet

Ellis, M. E. (2024, January 24). *Natural Relief from Arthritis Pain.* Health line. https://www.healthline.com/health/osteoarthritis/arthritis-natural-relief#diet

https://www.youtube.com/watch?v=M9F958Lgxec

Dr. Diana Girnita - Rheumatologist OnCall. (2023, October

13). *Natural remedies for rheumatoid arthritis pain relief* [Video]. YouTube. https://www.youtube.com/watch?v=M9F958Lgxec

46

About the Author

Meet Vandy,(Vandana Kapoor) an advocate for holistic well-being and the mind behind the upcoming book, HOME REME-DIES: **Natural Solutions for Everyday Wellness** .A passionate proponent of self-care and sustainable living, Vandy draws inspiration from traditional practices, blending ancient wisdom with modern lifestyles. Her mission is to empower readers to take charge of their health and wellness using easily accessible remedies found in their own homes.

Also by Vandana Kapoor

Vandana Kapoor is a dynamic individual with a passion for wildlife, financial markets, astrology, and wellness coaching. As a devoted wildlife enthusiast, she explores the wonders of nature, advocating for environmental conservation. Simultaneously, she navigates the intricate world of the stock market with analytical finesse. Embracing her fascination with the cosmos, She is also an adept astrologer, offering insights into celestial influences. Complementing her diverse interests, she serves as a wellness coach, guiding others toward holistic well-being. Her multifaceted journey is a vibrant tapestry of her diverse passions and expertise.

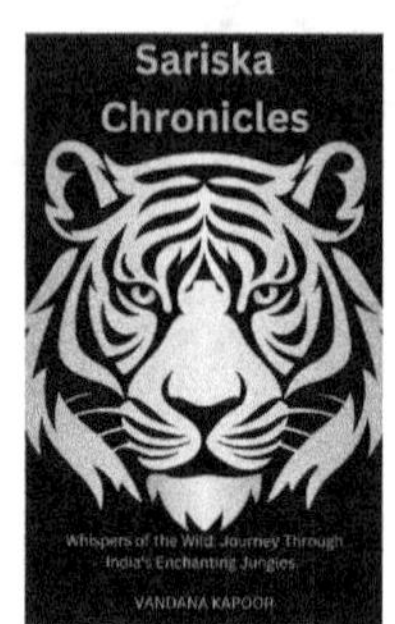

Sariska Chronicles

Sariska Chronicles invites you on an enchanting odyssey through the heart of India's wilderness. Uncover the secrets of Sariska Tiger Reserve Rajasthan ,India.Each page unfolds a tapestry of untamed beauty, majestic creatures, and the delicate dance between predator and prey. With a passion for wildlife as the guiding force, this chronicle unveils the mysteries of Sariska's mystical forests—a heartfelt tribute to the sanctuary's enduring allure and the captivating stories it holds.

www.ingramcontent.com/pod-product-compliance
Lightning Source LLC
Chambersburg PA
CBHW070726260726
48660CB00007B/2746

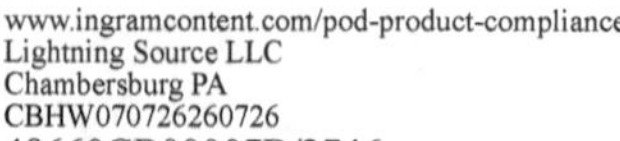